# Helping Your Spouse Beat Stage IV Cancer

The Never-Ending Cycle to Caregiving

Tracy Sparks

Copyright © Tracy Sparks, 2019

All rights reserved. No part of this book may be reproduced in any form without permission in writing from the author. Reviewers may quote brief passages in reviews.

Published 2019

DISCLAIMER

No part of this publication may be reproduced or transmitted in any form or by any means, mechanical or electronic, including photocopying or recording, or by any information storage and retrieval system, or transmitted by email without permission in writing from the author.

Neither the author nor the publisher assumes any responsibility for errors, omissions, or contrary interpretations of the subject matter herein. Any perceived slight of any individual or organization is purely unintentional.

Brand and product names are trademarks or registered trademarks of their respective owners.

*I thank my family for their love, guidance, and patience while I wrote this love letter to my caregiver family!*
*Here's to building more memories.*

# Table of Contents

Table of Contents ............................................. 4

Chapter 1: How am I supposed to do this? .. 6

Chapter 2: How I Went from Overwhelmed to Peace of Mind ................................................ 13

Chapter 3: How to Become a Caregiver ...... 28

Chapter 4: What Does the Diagnosis and Stage Mean? ................................................... 35

Chapter 5: Why Is It so Important to Find the Right Specialist? ........................................... 41

Chapter 6: What Are the Recommended Tests and Treatments? ................................. 48

Chapter 7: Why You May Need to Travel to Get the Best Medical Outcome .................... 58

Chapter 8: Working with Your Insurance Company ........................................................ 64

Chapter 9: Getting a Grip and Gaining Perspective .................................................... 71

Chapter 10: How Important Is It to Have a Support System? ......................................... 79

Chapter 11: A New Normal ........................... 89

Chapter 12: Where Do I Get the Strength to Take Care of Myself? ..................................... 94

Chapter 13: How Do I Handle the Most Difficult Days?............................................. 99

Chapter 14: Your Quality of Life ................. 107

About the Author ......................................... 112

Thank You .................................................... 114

# Chapter 1: How am I supposed to do this?

You may think that hearing your spouse having stage IV cancer is the worst news you can receive, until you realize you must be the person who cares for him. You must provide the stability that they will lack, their voice when they are not being heard, and the eyes and ears to make sure they are getting the best care they deserve.

It is up to you to make sure you are asking all the right questions at the right times. But you have questions of your own like:

- How am I supposed to do this?
- What if I can't do this?
- What happens if I get sick?
- Will I be able to find others to help me?
- How will I know what is the best care for my spouse?
- How expensive will this be?

- Can I continue to work and still address his needs?
- How do I tell our kids?
- Will he die?

You understand that this role is not a small one. There are many crucial moments you address delicately and some with more force. You also realize that it is not short-term. You see that every process is different and time-consuming. You educate yourself on not only the disease life expectancy but things like:

- How many surgeries has the doctor I picked done and what is his success rate?
- What does follow up treatment look like for this disease?
- Is it just scans, CT, PET, or MRI?
- Is it just bloodwork, tumor markers or CEA counts, or a combination of both or something completely different?
- Does this cancer fair well with chemo, radiation, both, and none?

- Is it one surgery, two, three, five, or seven?

As you know, there are many factors to be considered. Of course, keeping open communication with your spouse is just as important. They need to be aware of everything that is going on around them, even if they are sometimes bothered with all the information. Truly understanding and trying to meet their needs is beneficial to both of you.

You move through this journey numb and raw all at the same time. You hear words you do not know the meaning of, you cannot pronounce, and just seem made up. You are confused through most of the process, especially because you are so emotionally attached to the patient. All of this is okay! Yes, it is *okay!* You are human! You are learning a lot about yourself. You find the strength within yourself that you never thought you had. You tackle so many tasks that there are days you feel like Superman! You also have many days where you don't feel like getting out of bed. You develop patterns and get into routines once you receive the diagnosis and stage. Getting into your groove serves you both well.

Diagnosis and stage is defined and redefined along your journey. These are a few pieces of a lengthy process you need to know to move forward in getting the right care for your loved one. It is not just one of the components that matter. It is a combination of them that make the process work, work well, and be extremely efficient. There is unfortunately not much time to stop and smell the roses when a stage IV diagnosis is heard. It is important to research, but it needs to be done correctly. Focusing on the bad, the negative, and the sad outcomes will only keep you frozen in time. That surely is not in your or your spouse's best interest. Having gone through this myself I had many failures and many successes. I was able to make my husband maintain his weight during chemotherapy just by incorporating a few herbs and supplements into a smoothie. He experienced neuropathy during chemotherapy which only allowed him to eat and drink room temperature foods and drinks. I learned many tricks to allow him to still feel his independence as he attempted to conquer the refrigerator or freezer or drink a cup of hot tea. I added different strengths of CBD oils and treatments to his existing regimens. I helped my husband and many others throughout our journey find the right combination for many of these tasks. Throughout chemotherapy I would sit with other families and help research their specific diagnosis, help with healthcare plans, find world renowned surgeons, make phone calls for clinical trials, and talk with them about taking care of themselves as the caregiver. It is essential to create stability and stay well balanced from diagnosis to recovery. I am honored to have helped many families throughout their cancer journeys but am thankful corporations are recognizing caregivers in a different manner.

There has been a major focus on caregivers in the past year. Companies are realizing the important role we play and are offering more options than in previous years. In 2019, GuideWell launched a $400,000 Caring for Caregivers Innovation Challenge. It is focused on addressing critical barriers family caregivers face while caring for adult family members. They will award the money to four companies or non-profit organizations with sustainable, innovative approaches to reduce or eliminate the complex issues faced by family caregivers every day. Applicants will be evaluated on their ability to develop and deploy approaches that support the mental, social, and economic health of family caregivers and improve their ability to care for loved ones. The focus will be on providing affordable, accessible solutions that improve the quality of life for family caregivers, the loved ones they are caring for, and other family members living in the same home as the caregiver.

Also, many corporations are adding a Caregiver Leave Program to their benefits packages. A Florida company will introduce the caregiver benefit to their employees. This company recognizes the importance of family to employees and is offering a two-week (eighty hours) paid caregiver leave program beginning January 1, 2020. It is designed to support employees when they need time away to care for an immediate family member suffering from a serious health condition. Eligible employees must first qualify for Family Medical Leave (FMLA) which will run concurrently with the two-week, paid

Caregiver Leave Program. They are compensated at 100 percent of their base pay.

Regardless of how overwhelming this feels, getting over the shock of the diagnosis is just the beginning of this long journey! You can do this! It takes some getting used to with new schedules, introducing new medications and treatments, and learning how to be present for your spouse, your family, your friends, and yourself. When you help to provide the best care, options, and resources and operate as a team, it becomes the most important and critical way to navigate through becoming the best caregiver.

# Chapter 2: How I Went from Overwhelmed to Peace of Mind

My role as a caregiver to my extremely healthy fifty-one-year-old husband began in May of 2018. It was not something I ever saw coming, and I always thought if anyone would get sick, it would be his chubby wife with three kids who doesn't like to exercise and enjoys her ice cream sundaes a little too much! All joking aside, I was feeling beat-up, defeated, pissed-off, and scared. I thought, "I am a good person; why is this happening to my family?!" I never pictured being widowed at forty-seven years old. I was married young and thought I would have a forever companion.

You never quite recover from hearing the news. It's like you remember so vividly in your mind where you were, how you sat, where the doctor stood, the reaction on the nurse's face, and the drop in your chest. The sad feelings you felt for your husband, wondering what he must be feeling and thinking while receiving this news. Then, you begin to wonder if he knows there is nothing that you won't do to get him better!

My husband argued with me and his family doctor about getting a routine colonoscopy done because he turned fifty. He was never overweight and was the guy most people would ask for help. His favorite expression was, "I train for this!"

He started with an at-home test that came back positive. He called me from an airport terminal wondering if he should be concerned. I instantly googled, "What does a positive Cologuard result mean?" Even though it said many report false positives, we knew scheduling an appointment to get a colonoscopy was the right thing to do. We had just moved from New York to Georgia, so we were still establishing new doctors.

It took me three months to get a new patient appointment with my primary doctor. She was gracious enough to squeeze my husband in on one of her half-days because she sensed the urgency in my voice. She referred him to a gastroenterologist and met two weeks later. Since his medical history showed no signs for concern, we were confident it is just a false positive. We arrived at the appointment for the colonoscopy and I signed all the necessary paperwork since I was driving him home. I was called back by a nurse to wait in the recovery room until he woke up. I am a people-watcher, so I watched the doctor visiting each patient and telling them to get dressed, that they were free to leave. I expected the same process for us, but before he came to our door, he stopped at the nurse's station and grabbed a chair. The doctor came in, saying words that for some reason I could not string together. I had heard them, but they never pertained to anyone in my family!

I was overwhelmed. I had said, *"What!* You said a mass?"

"Yes, I did," he said.

"But you said cancer?" I asked.

He said, "Yes, I did. A mass *is* cancer."

I did not know this...or maybe I did. I was so confused! I was alone in a room where when my spouse wakes up from the anesthesia, I have to tell that he has cancer. **And I thought my only role that**

**morning was to provide transportation for this procedure!**

He did not wake up groggily like they said he would, so I had to share the news. It took all I had in me to tell him to not worry and that we were going to beat this. Of course, he was in shock. I told him I had already begun my research to find out what this entails. We were not given a lot of information except that more tests would need to be run to confirm pathology. That would take three to six days. I started to think about how I was going to tell our kids and family. We discussed it and decided to just tell the kids for now. We would tell family on a need-to-know basis.

The pathology came back and it confirmed it was colon cancer. I googled "life expectancy" even though I knew I shouldn't. We all do!!! We needed to move forward in finding a surgeon. I asked a woman in the waiting room where my husband was having a CT scan if she had any recommendations for local surgeons. Her dad had bone cancer. We shared our stories and embraced because we both understood what it felt like to be so helpless. She offered up a great recommendation. We picked the surgeon that was recommended. He was older but very well experienced.

The CT scan results showed that cancer had not metastasized. Woo-hoo! We celebrated this small victory.

We had plans to attend my niece's wedding out of state, but surgery was scheduled for the following Monday. A two-day cleanse is required, so we needed to inform our family. This was tough! I argued with my parents in January. I had not talked to them much since our argument. Also, my husband had not had a relationship with his family in years. *You must tell your family that your husband has cancer, right? That is the proper thing to do.*

I decided to tell my sister and her husband first. It was very heartbreaking. My sister offered to tell my parents and I focused on preparing my husband for surgery.

His right hemicolectomy surgery had started. It would take one-and-a-half hours, and they would remove his cecum, appendix, some lymph nodes and parts of his colon and intestines. When surgery was complete, my kids and I headed back to a room to talk with the doctor. He mentioned words like, a peritoneum lining, HIPEC, and cytoreductive surgery. *What?* He said he did not think we were dealing with colon cancer anymore. *Wait* – not again! He said he thinks it is appendix cancer, but we would have to wait for pathology. My next thought was, "An appendix, this can't be so bad – people get those removed all the time" Well, I was wrong, *again!* After I googled appendix cancer, I saw the very grim outcomes and was informed that if it spread from the place of origin, it was Stage IV. This is the only time you should be allowed to google anything medical. You can find out definitions but not life expectancies; that information only makes you feel more defeated. If we trusted the life expectancies statistics, he would have been dead in less than ten months. Appendix cancer is rare and hard to diagnose. We were lucky to have had a surgeon who was knowledgeable about other types of cancers. He knew something looked different and took steps to remove most of the disease. This is now *the second time* I am left to tell my husband after gaining consciousness that he has something different. He would wake up now having Stage IV appendix cancer. I love rollercoasters, but this ride had to end!

Our next step was to look for a local oncologist to start chemotherapy. He needed another small surgery to put the port in to receive the chemo treatments. His previous surgeon was able to perform this day surgery. We also needed to find a surgical oncologist to perform his HIPEC surgery. After visiting a few places, we settled on North Carolina. If this was his best chance at beating this disease, then that is where we would go. I wanted him to know how much I supported him, and we would travel anywhere to get the best care and outcome.

We met with the wonderful staff who explained the procedure. They said,

*It will be between a six to twenty-four-hour surgery.*

*We will start laparoscopically and take out everything we see that is diseased.*

*I will not know the true amount of disease until I open you up.*

*We will run hot chemo through your stomach cavity for ninety minutes; if we can even get to this step depending on the severity of the disease.*

*I will not know if chemo will be required after the surgery until I look at what is inside.*

*We will schedule surgery one month after your last round of chemo."*

Well, that is a lot of information, but it isn't at all very specific!!

How could I handle not having any answers until that moment?

How was I supposed to receive news sitting in another waiting room after he has surgery?

*What if there is more bad news to tell him when he wakes up?*

He needs the surgery to survive so we will deal with whatever comes our way!

Chemotherapy went better than I had anticipated. That's according to me, I am sure my husband has a different perspective considering I was just there to watch and support. We did six rounds every other week. It ran from August through October. In between that time, we had to deal with low white blood cell counts and shots to boost them. We met many great people. Some of them were fighting alone! I promised myself I would enter each appointment with a smile on my face, even though it is the saddest place I have seen in my lifetime. These patients are hopeful! They are fighting for their lives! They are hanging on by a thread but show up each time looking to be cured. They were the humblest people I have met. No one was bitter or lived their life with regrets. They saw the positive in everything, even during the most negative time in their lives.

Some days the patients in chemotherapy would crave fast food. Another caregiver and I would run through a few drive-thru's and purchase some burgers and fries. They were so thankful, and we were delighted just knowing we were able to provide a little happiness in that moment.

His big day was approaching! We arrived the day before his surgery for pretesting. My family and friends were there. His mother, brother, and sister were there too. I kissed and hugged him before they wheeled him down the hallway. His family sat with mine. It was very awkward; even small talk was difficult. I kept the peace. I acted appropriately, and when the time came for the doctor to explain what happened in surgery, I allowed them to attend. The doctor said he had limited disease. This is the best news we had heard so far! I am also proud of myself for handling our family issues with such grace.

My husband was brought back to his room, and I could not help but think about what he had gone through. In just six short months, he had three surgeries, six rounds of intravenous chemo, many shots to boost his white blood cell count, HIPEC, seen two doctors, one surgeon, one oncologist, one surgical oncologist, and never had pain, or any symptom before the diagnosis...crazy!

While my husband was recovering, I found out through my online support group, that another member was coming in for the same surgery. My family headed to her room to offer her support. We never met before, but we prayed with her for a successful surgery and recovery.

That evening, my husband had gone into AFib and was transferred to the ICU. It was scary, but the nurses reassured me he was there to be monitored due to the heart medication. We spent that night in the ICU. I tossed and turned, trying to get comfortable on the hospital chair.

I woke to use the serenity room. It is a room the hospital provides to caregivers who are there for long periods of time. I will never forget the moment I walked down that hallway and saw a hospital room filled with many doctors and nurses, blood everywhere, parents outside in the hallway talking to a surgeon. I listened quietly as I walked past. My new friend was bleeding from her liver, and they couldn't finish the surgery. They left her with an opened wound to allow her body to heal and try to stop the bleeding over the next day or so. I could not believe what I was hearing! This amazing person I met yesterday was going to die! No way! That could not happen! I walked back to our room and sobbed the entire night. I didn't cry this way over my husband's surgery but was so affected by someone I just met. I passed her room many times a day and prayed for her and her family, and I inwardly yelled at her to get back here because our relationship just began and she could not leave me! I checked on her like I said I would and continued to even when my husband was released from the ICU.

The doctors said my husband was recovering very well and he could get ready to go home. His mom, sister, and brother came by a few times to visit and sit with him while he was in the hospital. I stepped out of the room when they visited to allow them time to spend with him.

The day before he was going to be released, I noticed something wrong with myself. I just did not feel right. I tried walking, sitting, and even meditating, but nothing worked. I went outside to get some fresh air. I realized I had not left the hospital over the last ten days! The cool air on my face felt great. I didn't feel well enough to head back inside, so my dad and brother-in-law came to sit with my husband. The feelings I was having made me think I was going crazy, literally out of my mind. I felt weak and nauseous. My heart was racing. I knew logically what I was doing, but my brain could not keep up. I took a short nap and had a small meal and that made me feel better. My doctor later said that my body was crashing from the stress, lack of sleep, skipping meals, and concern for my husband. I had a great support system, and yet I still allowed this to happen!

He was released on day eleven. We stayed local for the next week for him to recover more and then drove the six hours back home. He was very uncomfortable and spent many days and nights in a recliner in the living room. He took his pain medication and antibiotics and I administered his anticoagulant shots. We only made two visits during his recovery to the ER due to medication issues.

Since it was almost holiday time, we decorated our house and followed all our normal traditions. We made him wear a light-up Christmas sweater as we took the fall decorations down and prepared for Christmas. We decorated our trees and wrapped presents. He was struggling both mentally and physically, though. He could not sit through an entire meal without having to get up to walk and stretch. Many times, at a restaurant, I was left alone to finish my meal as he headed out to the parking lot to walk. We incorporated chiropractic treatments and massage therapy into his recovery. That helped greatly, but you can see the pain in his eyes from the muscle spasms in his back and shoulders. He has lost thirty pounds already.

It was the first time I looked at him as a cancer patient. My heart always hurt for him, and I could not even envision what would go through his mind. I admit I also had many moments where I thought, "If cancer doesn't kill him, I will!" I had been at the end of my rope many times and had to bite my tongue more times than you could ever imagine. It's because cancer takes a toll on you and your family. It is hard to watch someone wither away. It is hard to tell him you are mad or upset. You don't want to complain about the rude cashier at Walmart or the driver in the car on Rt 17 that cut you off and almost totaled your car. You want to vent but realize that he is going through a lot and now is not the right time.

He returned to work full-time in February. We head to North Carolina every six months for a CT scan and bloodwork. So far, he is NED (No Evidence of Disease)! There are still many issues that can arise from a traumatic surgery and cancer diagnosis. At his last visit, the doctor said he has an incisional hernia.

That will require another surgery. When his CT scan was released from North Carolina to his current surgeon, I decided to "read" it. I noticed phrases like "thickening in an area" and "can't rule out recurrence." I felt my heart sink again. I immediately called his surgeon in North Carolina and asked why we were not told about this possible recurrence. He told me that I was reading a medical report that is only meant to be read between radiologists and surgeons. Radiologists document any changes from the last scan. "It does not mean it changed because cancer is present. It could change for many reasons," he said. "You need to remember that you are not his surgeon or radiologist and that he is in good hands."

With having appointments and scans every six months for the next ten years, I understand that I will always worry. I truly believe that I will ask him more frequently how he is feeling. Every time he complains something is hurting him, I will relate it to his cancer until I hear otherwise. I do believe however that if I am *all in* and continuously stay involved, it will always bring me the peace of mind that I need to continue to move forward.

# Chapter 3: How to Become a Caregiver

I often referred to my caregiving journey as being on a sailboat. I was riding on turbulent, stormy waters in the pouring down rain. I had wave after wave hitting me from every side. Many times, the boat seemed to rock to the point of flipping over, but somehow straightened itself out again. I had to figure out how to navigate, keep it stable, and when to raise my sails.

I remember thinking, "I am not a wife who holds a full-time job, and I am finding it difficult to take care of my spouse. I wonder how many wives are in the same situation as me, but they work full-time too." I first believed that I could handle this like a honey-do list. I could write down all my tasks and then check them off as I completed them. I soon learned that would not work. An example is when my husband was diagnosed with colon cancer. As I said in the last chapter, during the surgery he was having to remove the colon cancer, we found out it was appendix cancer. Therefore, this situation is not like your twelve-step program for AA that you can follow. It is an infinite loop; a never-ending cycle. I had to set parameters and create a framework that allowed me to process my thoughts, behaviors, and actions while I was experiencing many emotions at the same time.

Your journey will take you from diagnosis to treatment to survivorship, but there are many gray areas in between that will need to be addressed.

Here are my nine areas of interest in the cycle for caregiving:

1. Diagnosis and stage
2. Finding the right specialist
3. Recommended treatments and tests
4. Working with your insurance
5. Travel options
6. Getting a grip and gaining perspective
7. Having a support system
8. Your new normal
9. Taking care of yourself

**Diagnosis and stage** are your very first introduction to this disease. It is where you are the most surprised, shocked, and scared. It is where you will have the most questions because you recognize it is the earliest part of your long journey. You will research and google life expectancy because you think you want to know how long he will live. You will want to know if your children are now more susceptible to getting cancer.

**Finding the right specialist** is just as important because we feel once we narrowed down the diagnosis and stage, it will be simple to find the best surgeon. I found this difficult because you have opinions from friends, family members, and your doctor. Many observers can be adamant about who you should see. Keeping a clear mind and focusing on what is best for the patient will prove to be the most beneficial.

Next, there are many **tests and procedures** to help conquer this disease. There are scans, blood tests, surgeries, clinical trials, immunotherapy, and chemotherapy, just to name a few… some questions you may have are:

- What type of chemotherapy works for this disease?
- How will he react to this specific treatment?

- Does he meet all the criteria for this clinical trial?
- How many rounds of chemotherapy will he need?
- What if he is allergic to one, will we have to stop treatment or is there an alternative?
- What if he is not strong enough to handle the chemo or surgeries, will we have options?

**Contacting your insurance company** and getting answers could be one of the most difficult areas to navigate. Some hospitals require payment upfront before offering any services. Some locations will not accept your insurance. Many places will show you upfront what your costs will be. You may have insurance questions like:

- What is my deductible, copay and out of pocket expenses after treatments?
- Will my insurance cover the name brand medicines or generics?
- What if my insurance denies my life-saving surgeries?

**Travel options** are something I never thought we would have to address. I assumed all local oncologists handled all types of cancers. Many cancers can be addressed locally, but when you are diagnosed with a rare cancer, you may have to travel far to get the appropriate care. It could be a matter of life and death! Some major corporations are starting to offer a new travel benefit for any cancer diagnosis, regardless of their local options. This is another area to research.

Another area of interest is taking an intimate approach to help you stay close to your spouse by **getting a grip and gaining perspective**. It gives ideas on how to stay connected and how to communicate through this difficult time. When I was able to ask my husband a question and understand his answer, it made an impact on how I continued with his care.

**Your support system** can be your family, your friends, your Facebook posts, or even your dog! I would recommend all of them and finding an online or local organization specific to your spouse's disease. There are spousal support programs, cancer support programs, and specific disease programs like ACPMP or PMP Pals for appendix cancer patients and caregivers. Being able to talk about successes and failures can provide you with the extra support you need.

**Your new normal** may not be what you are thinking. Do you remember your kid's move-in day freshman year in college? You had to rearrange your schedule that weekend to make sure you allowed yourself enough time to move them in, grocery shop, take them for dinner before you left, and allow time for the many tears that were shed. Or the time when your spouse was home sick from work and you had to handle all the responsibilities for that day like chauffeuring the kids to practice, laundry, and preparing dinner. Your new normal is…*change.* It may feel a little different, but it is addressed the same way you would handle all the other changes in your life.

**Taking care of myself** is one I found most difficult. I learned over the years that I am not the type of woman who puts herself first. I have stayed home raising my kids. They were always my priority.

Next was my husband, family, and friends. I did not know how to put myself first. I always heard that if you don't take care of yourself, you cannot care for others. Put your oxygen mask on first. I got this concept, I just struggled with incorporating it into my life. I felt selfish if I told others no, especially if I was doing something for myself. But I soon learned how important it was to **find my own caregiver.** You need to look out for yourself due to the stress you endure throughout this journey.

Remember that your goal is to get your spouse to NED or cured from cancer. You can do this by using the nine areas of interest simultaneously and by allowing yourself the space you need to think logically and make those important decisions for your loved one.

One of my favorite quotes that sums up my feelings on being a caregiver says, "Remember that you cannot change the direction of the wind but you can adjust your sails to always reach your destination!"

# Chapter 4: What Does the Diagnosis and Stage Mean?

## Diagnosis:

The National Institute of Health defines family caregiving as unpaid assistance to family members who are unable to function independently. It's an important component of care for family members who are terminally ill, severely disabled, or have chronic conditions such as memory disorders, cancer, strokes, or pulmonary diseases.

According to the National Alliance for Caregiving, there were more than 43.5 million adults in the U.S. who provided unpaid care to a family member in 2015. I fall into the 34.2 million who care for a senior family member aged fifty or older.

Your spouse will be dealing with many emotions when he is first diagnosed. You will also be dealing with your own emotions. The sooner you start to deal with them, the quicker you will lower your stress levels and improve your mental, physical, and emotional health. Try surrounding yourself with people who are positive and happy to be around. You will begin to gain more confidence and a greater sense of hope while you work through the progression of the disease. If you ever feel like you are not able to get through this, please do not hesitate to seek medical attention. Depression is a very serious illness and there are many medications and counseling available, so you do not have to go through this alone.

People who provide long term care for a chronically ill family member face many challenges within their daily lives. These challenges include stress and burnout, financial burdens, career sacrifices, sleep deprivation, depression, isolation, and lack of privacy. On average, a family caregiver will spend more than twenty-four hours each week providing care to a loved one, and seventy-five percent of these family caregivers are also working.

Diagnosis consists of many areas. There are many teaching hospitals throughout the country and a handful of world-renowned surgical oncologists that can help with a rare diagnosis. Some tests to determine diagnosis are not very accurate. Some rare cancers are hard to detect on any scans and they do not show any symptoms prior to diagnosis. A surgical oncologist described why it is so hard to detect rare cancers on a scan. A regular cancer tumor would look like a grape, so if you scanned that area, it would show up with a grape-sized lump in that specific area. With some rare cancers it would be like taking thirty grapes squashing and smearing them into the same area where that lump should be, making it nearly undetectable. That is why it is impossible to know how much disease is present. Also, diagnosis is not always associated with demographics or it being hereditary. In some cases, children or immediate family members would not have to be tested any earlier for certain cancers and while in other cases they do not even have a test for it!

Even though a diagnosis is established, there are still so many unanswered questions.

## Stage:

Cancer consists of a group of more than 100 variations. It is important to know the specific type of cancer your spouse has been diagnosed with to move forward with treatment options. There are many diagnostic tests doctors use to determine cancer's stage. Staging is used to describe where cancer might be in the body. It can also tell if or where it has spread and if it is affecting other areas of the body. The stages range from 0-IV.

Stage 0 is when the cancer is still located in the place of origin and has not spread to nearby tissues. It is often highly curable and requires surgery to remove the entire tumor.

Stage I is when a tumor has not grown into the tissues too deeply. It has not spread to lymph nodes or other areas in the body.

Stage II and III are larger cancers that grew deeper into the tissues. They could have spread to lymph nodes but not any organs.

Stage IV is when it has spread to other organs and areas of the body. It is usually referred to as advanced or metastatic cancer.

We battled Stage IV. We did not know what this meant given there are varying degrees in Stage IV. Not all Stage IV diagnosis are equal. Some diagnosis has multiple options, and some are limited to just palliative and home care. We had one recommended medical option. We always had a plan and that kept us focused on what was next versus reflecting on what the doctor had just told us. Hearing Stage IV would make anyone feel helpless and defeated. Our middle daughter came to this appointment. She had one year left until she became a chiropractor and offered her advice and support. It was comforting having her there to be an extra set of ears, especially during such an emotional visit. I did ask how much time my husband had left. The oncologist said, "I do not know because he can walk out of here today and get hit by a bus." I cried on the way home.

It was the only time during this journey that I felt afraid and lost. I did not know enough about this disease and how to beat it. I promised myself that I would not feel that way again. I would educate myself to the point of being confident to ask any questions, to not be afraid to say if I did not understand, and to continue to dig deep into the new advances to beat this beast of a disease.

This area of interest will be challenging but don't get lost in the Stage. Remember this is the way the medical community breaks down diagnosis of cancer and how they approach defining treatment options.

The important part for you as a caregiver is to understand all your options, what questions to ask, and to stay focused on what lies ahead.

# Chapter 5: Why Is It so Important to Find the Right Specialist?

In 2019, a cancer patient experience survey was conducted. One question asked, "Which resources do patients use when deciding where to go for their care?" *Eighty-one percent* of patients said they consulted their primary doctor. Another question was, "What is your preferred level of control when making decisions about your cancer treatment?" *Fifty percent* responded, "My doctor and I make the decisions together."

I have a concern about this survey. Some primary care physicians do not know enough about certain cancers and other diseases to direct their patients. I worry that the patient will not take the necessary time to research and just use their doctor's recommendations. As a caregiver, it is very important to do your due diligence. I developed a set of questions based on my research and discussed it with our doctor. I understood there may be options out there that even he did not know about. Two of my questions were:

> 1. Have you had other patients with this specific disease who you referred to this surgeon?
> 2. What were their outcomes?

It is a reasonable expectation that your doctor would tell you he does not have a very good understanding of this disease and would only expect that you will investigate other options.

We visited a very prestigious teaching hospital through a recommendation from our local oncologist. At the time, we thought this is where my husband would have his CRS/HIPEC surgery. I went in with a clear head and an open mind. I paid close attention to how their offices operated and their timeliness. My reason for doing this was because I knew we would be spending weeks at this facility and with this staff.

It seemed many patients kept asking the receptionist when they would be seen after they had been there for quite some time. The surgery can take all day, and I wanted to feel as comfortable with my surroundings as he was with receiving the proper care. They took us to our 12:30 p.m. appointment at 3:30 p.m. After reviewing my husband's records, the doctor announced that she was not very familiar with this type of appendix cancer. She has done many CRS/HIPEC surgeries for colon and ovarian cancer, but not appendix.

My husband's cancer is non-mucinous. They described it as if cancer "flakes" off and attaches itself to the lymph nodes, organs, or into the bloodstream. It is a silent killer because there are no symptoms before diagnosis. Many patients are diagnosed at stage IV. The non-mucinous type can respond to systemic chemotherapy.

Based on a variety of factors but mostly my gut feeling, I knew we would not be having HIPEC surgery there. Trust your instincts!

We consulted with our local oncologist and explained why we did not use his recommendation. We needed to find a place where we felt comfortable in their abilities to tackle this rare disease. He only encouraged us to keep looking to find the right fit. Many specialists know how vulnerable and helpless you feel, and they should encourage you to look outside their referral if needed. They realize you need them to help you make some serious life decisions.

Another important question asked through this survey was, "Which features are most important to patients when deciding where to go for care?" The top answer was to a doctor who specializes in their cancer.

I wish many caregivers could know how critical this is. I understand the immense pressure you are already under and you are trying to juggle your responsibilities. A local doctor may not be able to handle your spouse's diagnosis. Remember, there are many areas to explore. You can focus on the holistic approach. Nutrition, exercise, massage, and chiropractic care are just a few examples. You can choose the medical approach, or you can incorporate both. Investigate thoroughly. I have noticed too many times patients limiting themselves to certain care. For any rare cancer, it is crucial to get checked quickly and set up a treatment plan. There are also certain criteria you need to meet to qualify for the surgery. It depends on your health for your age, your lifestyle before surgery, and your mental outlook on life. Some patients who wait too long are not able to have life-saving surgery because their cancer has progressed. Just keep your focus on the best care for your loved one.

In the same survey, they asked, "Why did you change cancer care providers?" *Twenty-eight percent* answered, "I found a different doctor who specializes in my care."

A specialist can truly make a difference between life and death. When someone new joins my appendix cancer support group and begins to ask questions, the very first response is, "Do you have an appendix cancer specialist?" At first, it surprised me how many people would pose that question. Then, with further understanding of this disease, I realized how very crucial that question (and response) was. Some appendix cancer patients needed three CRS/HIPEC surgeries and are still here to tell their amazing story! Even if you have a recurrence, you are still being monitored by a professional who can act quickly and appropriately and together you can move forward understanding the best options for your treatment plan.

I am very aware of the impact on the caregiver when your specialist is not local. A friend of mine was diagnosed with a rare cancer on the west coast many years ago and decided to have her appointments at a local prestigious hospital. When she met with the surgeon, he told her to not get her hopes up because many patients die soon from this disease. He also said if they don't die from that they will die because most insurance companies will decline your claim. She refused to have her surgery performed there. She researched and found a newspaper article rating the top ten doctors for her rare cancer. She wrote each of them a handwritten note and mailed it to their offices. Everyone but one got back with her by calling her at her home. The doctor she chose on the east coast to perform her surgery was the one who asked her to forward her records directly to him. He later called her to read them out loud to her and explain exactly what type and stage of cancer she had.

Knowing how to find the perfect specialist can take some work but it is doable. Leverage all your resources, talk to your doctors, engage your support groups and do your homework. Remember the more informed you are about your decision, the better you will feel in the end.

# Chapter 6: What Are the Recommended Tests and Treatments?

From diagnosis to full recovery, you will be researching many tests that need to be performed. You will also research the best treatments and what procedures there are for your specific disease. You will be asking questions at every level and gathering your results to move forward. Some of the questions asked here will be:

- Why is this test so important?
- What are we looking to find when administering this test?
- What are our alternatives and options if this test comes back positive?

If you are lucky, you will have many treatment options. You want as many viable options as possible. When you are limited on options is when the disease has progressed to a point where they cannot be of much assistance.

Our journey started by having an at-home test. They measure if there is any blood or DNA in your stool. It is not 100 percent accurate and should only be used by people who do not have any prior gastrointestinal issues or are recommended by your primary care physician.

A colonoscopy is usually the next recommended test. It is an outpatient procedure in which the inside of the large intestine (colon and rectum) is examined. A colonoscopy is commonly used to evaluate gastrointestinal symptoms, such as rectal and intestinal bleeding or changes in bowel habits. It is performed by a doctor experienced in the procedure and lasts approximately thirty to sixty minutes. Medications are given intravenously to make you feel relaxed and drowsy. The doctor is looking for any abnormalities in the colon. There is a prep required before the test to clean out the colon. You will need someone to drive you home from this procedure since you are under sedation. Recovery is very basic with rest and a light diet. During the colonoscopy, they reach an area called the cecum. The cecum is an intraperitoneal pouch that is the beginning of the large intestine. It is typically located on the right side of the body (the same side of the body as the appendix, to which it is joined). It receives undigested food material from the small intestine.

A CT (computed tomography) scan with contrast, also called a CAT scan, is the next test. This is a scan with a special dye called contrast that is administered intravenously to help highlight the areas of your body being examined. The contrast material blocks x-rays and appears white on images, which can help emphasize blood vessels, intestines, or other structures. The test itself takes only fifteen to thirty minutes performed in a hospital's radiology department or a clinic that specializes in diagnostic procedures. CT scans can show a tumor's shape, size, and location. They can even show the blood vessels that feed the tumor-all without having to cut into the patient. By comparing CT scans done over time, doctors can see how a tumor is responding to treatment or find out if cancer has come back after treatment.

A general surgeon performs a right hemicolectomy. It is a type of surgery done to remove part of your large intestine called your colon. Your colon could be partially removed without affecting the way it works in your digestive system. During a hemicolectomy, only one side of the colon is removed. The side of the colon removed depends on the location of the tumor or diseased intestine. It can be performed either laparoscopically or using open surgery. The transverse colon is then attached to the small intestine. There is preoperative testing to make sure you are an appropriate candidate. It includes an EKG (electrocardiogram) and blood tests. You have another bowel cleansing prep for two days before surgery. It is recommended post-surgery to eat certain foods to help control bowel movements like applesauce, yogurt, bananas, and high-fiber foods. They also recommend drinking more water.

In our situation, this surgeon found more disease than he expected when he operated. He mentioned that he removed much more of the colon than he had anticipated and scraped my husband's peritoneum lining and part of his small intestine. He also mentioned that the next surgery would remove all the lingering cancer cells. He sent biopsies out to the lab and we waited on a new diagnosis.

It came back as stage IV adenocarcinoma ex-goblet cell (GCC). It is a rare tumor normally occurring in the appendix which displays features of both neuroendocrine tumors and a more aggressive form of cancer known as adenocarcinoma. It is usually diagnosed in people over the age of fifty. My husband was fifty-one at diagnosis. In general, seventy-six percent of individuals who are diagnosed with GCC live at least five years after being diagnosed. The most important factors to consider when determining prognosis include the size and location of the tumor and whether cancer has spread to other parts of the body. If cancer cells have spread to distant parts of the body, the chances of survival are decreased.

We met with the general surgeon again to insert a port-a-cath. It is also referred to as a port. It is an implanted device that allows easy access to a patient's veins. It is surgically inserted completely beneath the skin and consists of two parts – the portal wand and the catheter. The portal is typically made from a silicone bubble and appears as a small bump under the skin. The portal, made of special self-sealing silicone, can be punctured by a needle repeatedly before the strength of the material is compromised. Its design contributes to a very low risk of infection. The slender plastic catheter attached to the portal is threaded into a central vein (usually the jugular or subclavian vein). His surgery took less than an hour. Recovery took a few days. They were able to administer chemo through this port in his chest.

Chemotherapy was next. Chemotherapy is the use of drugs to destroy cancer cells, usually by ending the cancer cell's ability to grow and divide. For appendix cancer that is not a neuroendocrine tumor, chemotherapy is most often used soon after surgery when cancer is found outside the appendix region. It is administered by a medical oncologist.

There are different types of chemotherapy. One is systemic and the other is local/intraperitoneal. This treatment gets into the bloodstream to reach cancer cells throughout the body. There are specific drugs given. My husbands were Folfox and Oxaliplatin. The side effects he experienced were nausea, loss of appetite, neuropathy, and hair thinning.

Neupogen shots had to be administered throughout his chemotherapy sessions. It may help the body make white blood cells after receiving cancer medications. It can also improve survival in people who have been exposed to radiation. You can experience bone pain with these shots. Claritin was administered to lessen the pain.

His last surgery to date was CRS/HIPEC. HIPEC is also known as heated or hyper thermic intraperitoneal chemotherapy. It is the process of heating chemotherapy drugs and delivering them into the abdominal cavity. This treatment is often combined with cytoreductive surgery where doctors remove visible tumors within the abdomen. HIPEC is circulated throughout the abdomen for approximately one-and-a-half hours at over 105 degrees Fahrenheit. It is possible for HIPEC to completely cure twenty-five to thirty percent of patients with certain types of cancers.

During his recovery from CRS/HIPEC, he visited a chiropractor and massage therapist three times a week for six weeks. This along with his medical care helped him heal quicker. It allowed him to re-strengthen his posture and to massage scar tissue that appeared from a long surgery.

A CT scan and bloodwork is required every six months until he reaches a five-year mark of being NED. Then he will go yearly for five more years. A radiologist reads the CT scans and documents any changes no matter how small. This allows them to see any progression over time.

A tumor marker may help to diagnose cancer, plan treatment, find out how well treatment is working or if cancer has come back. An example is CEA in colon cancer. A tumor marker is a substance found in tissue, blood or other body fluids that may be a sign of cancer or certain noncancer conditions. In my husband's case, his tumor markers never fluctuated so we now rely on scans to help monitor for recurrence.

Around nine months after surgery, my husband decided to remove his port. It is removed using local anesthesia. This is done in an operating room. During the procedure, a small incision is made, and the port and catheter are removed. The wound is closed with steristrips.

Incisional hernias are common after this type of surgery. It is a protrusion of tissue that forms at the site of a healing surgical scar. Incisional hernias do not heal on their own and require surgical treatment to repair. The surgery consists of pushing the protruding tissue back in place, removing any scar tissue, and adhering a surgical mesh on the hernia opening to prevent a recurrence. It can be done laparoscopically, and general anesthesia is typically used. Depending on the size of the hernia and the complexity of the surgery, patients are either released the same day or stay overnight in the hospital. We have our first surgeon consultation at the end of this week. We have moved since he had his previous surgeries, so we are starting the interviewing of doctors all over again to find who fits our new needs.

I recently followed a thread through my support group. A new patient asked if a surgery was worth having. She had mentioned most people have major complications following such a brutal surgery and is debating on whether she would subject her body to it. To date, 400 patients responded saying they would take the after-effects of the surgery over not having the surgery at all. Some reasons they listed were, "I got to see my grandson get married," "I lived to see my daughter graduate from her doctorate," and "I traveled to many places that I never imagined I would go."

In our situation, we never argued about the process for tests and treatments needed. We made sure to ask the necessary questions associated with each procedure. We knew this was the best way to better understand the disease and then decide how we would move forward with treatment options.

# Chapter 7: Why You May Need to Travel to Get the Best Medical Outcome

Sometimes, we feel like we trust our primary care physician so much that we need to listen to everything they say. That is why some people pick them. We continue to see our primary care physician because we feel like they have our best interests in mind. We really should be talking openly with our physician and deciding together what our next steps will be.

My husband and I grew up in a small town in Pennsylvania. We moved to upstate New York when my husband graduated with his MBA and accepted a job with a Fortune 100 company. I, of course, was worried about finding a great school for my kids to attend, finding a pediatrician's office, and making new friends. What I loved about my hometown was that I trusted my doctors and already created a rapport with them. . Moving just a few short hours away, I realized that I had to find new doctors to trust. I got pregnant with our third child, so I also had to find an OBGYN who met our needs. It was easy when I lived back home. My doctor was my doctor because my aunt worked in his office. My dentist was my dentist because my dad knew him from high school. My chiropractor was my cousin. No brainer for sure!

After 18 years in upstate NY, we decided to move south because of the warmer winters. We settled on Georgia and made it our home for the next four years. This was where my husband was diagnosed with appendix cancer. This was where we needed to find a general surgeon, an oncologist, and an appendix cancer specialist very soon! I immediately started checking local doctors.

I remember when I lived back home, my friend's father was sick. He had a rare form of cancer. His wife would take him to Philadelphia to be seen by specialists. When Philadelphia could not help him because they were not familiar with that type of cancer, she brought him home and he was admitted to hospice and palliative care. They gave them other locations like Texas and Arizona where they had experience with his condition, but he did not want to travel outside their state.

Just a few years ago, my parents decided to retire to Orlando, Florida. My parents lived in their hometown from birth to their mid-sixties. They had the same doctors and medical professionals for years. When they finally found a primary care physician they liked, they made an appointment. My dad had already been on high blood pressure pills, depression medication, and cholesterol pills. The doctor did some routine blood work and ran a few tests. My dad's triglycerides were high and his thyroid levels were off. She asked if he had ever been tested for these or if he was ever on any medication for them. He said he had known for years his triglycerides were high but knew nothing about his thyroid. His blood work showed he was diabetic. She started him on triglyceride, thyroid, and diabetic medication. He has lost twenty pounds to date and looks and feels better than ever. It's not that his primary care physician in Pennsylvania was a bad doctor. Nor do I feel that he did not take care of my dad. I feel that when you get into a routine, you may not want to complain or ask questions. You feel the doctor knows you and you trust them. I think we still need to realize that this is about our health. You have every right to ask questions, research many places, and then head back to your doctor to discuss. Many of your appointments can be handled locally. It is when you get a rare diagnosis that you need to rethink your options.

The healthcare industry is picking up on the need to work with the right specialist. A report in the Wall Street Journal mentioned that to reduce health spending while receiving quality care, companies such as Amazon, Lowe's, McKesson, and Walmart would pay for their employees with cancer to travel to "centers of excellence." They also pay for lodging expenses. It is a travel option that is provided through their benefits package for any cancer diagnosis, regardless of their local options. Their programs are designed so the patient has access to the individualized treatments as early as possible to help ensure the correct care is administered first. Companies can get more competitive pricing and employees receive better care. It avoids unnecessary treatment by having nationwide options rather than relying just on local providers.

I am happy I was allowed to move to upstate New York, Florida, and Georgia. I could not have guessed at the knowledge it would provide me in making the best caretaking travel decisions for my husband by taking the time to research the facility, the doctors, the location, and the patient and caregiver reviews. Sometimes we get stuck, possibly complacent when we grew up and lived forever in one place. Maybe we are scared and do not know if we can take the risk and try another facility farther away, especially when we are dealing with sickness where you need the most support. It is not unreasonable to think about how you will do it alone. I cannot say for sure that if I still lived up north when my husband got diagnosed that I would stay local or still research another location. I know there are many great treatment facilities in Buffalo, New York and New York City but the right fit for us was in Wake Forest, North Carolina. I hope that I have developed solid relationships with my physicians in New York and that they would work with me on getting the best care for my husband. I just doubt myself since I like a safe place and enjoy feeling the love of having my family and friends so close.

    I am proud of myself for how I handled our situation. I am proud of all the research that I did and continue to do to make sure my husband gets the best care. Remember to keep an open mind and don't let the location of care change your approach.

# Chapter 8: Working with Your Insurance Company

Insurance companies can be very intimidating. There is so much information you need to know, especially when you are dealing with a rare disease. There are also many factors when care is provided in different states. Here are a few questions you may have:

- What does deductible mean in insurance terms?

A deductible refers to the amount of money you must pay from your pocket every year before you can enjoy the benefits of your insurance plan. Deductibles are commonly confused with other out-of-pocket payments such as co-payments and co-insurance.

- What is a copay?

A copay (short for copayment) is a monetary charge that your health insurance plan may require you to pay to receive a specific medical service or supply. For example, your health insurance plan may require a $15 copay for an office visit or brand-name prescription drugs.

- What does the term coinsurance mean?

Coinsurance is a term that indicates the percentage of a covered service that you're responsible for. For example, if your medical insurance plan says your coinsurance for a CT scan is twenty percent, you're expected to pay twenty percent of the cost of your CT scan.

- Can you explain the out-of-pocket limit?

An out-of-pocket limit (or out-of-pocket maximum) is the maximum amount of money you may pay for medical services in a calendar year. Out-of-pocket limit may and may not include a deductible depending on insurers' definition of the term.

Health insurance coverage typically covers most doctors and hospital visits, prescription drugs, well-care, and medical devices. What health insurance does not cover:

- Most will not cover elective or cosmetic procedures, beauty

treatments, off-label drug use, or brand-new technologies
- If coverage is denied, policyholders can appeal for exemptions or allowances based on an individual's situation and prognosis
- Some doctors' offices will help consumers navigate through the insurance issues to determine coverage; however, as a consumer, it is recommended that you speak directly with the insurance company to confirm that the procedure is covered.
  - Despite this recommendation, insurance companies will sometimes only speak with the physician's office but persistence generally pays off

Some other common terms are:
- Pre-approval is one area of importance to pay attention to, as many insurance plans require it for procedures.

- In-network vs. out of network: many insurance plans are designed with in-network doctors and facilities. These in-network providers often have a contract negotiated with the insurance company to pay an agreed-upon price for various services. Ensure that all areas for a procedure are covered. For example, check that not only a surgeon and the hospital are in-network, but also the anesthesiologist. Make sure the tests are sent to an in-network lab.
- The cost and coverage of prescription drugs vary, depending on the plan's formulary. The formulary, typically found on a health insurer's website, details cheaper drugs via tier 1 versus tier 3, substitutes, or generic versions of the drugs. Also, some specialty drugs, such as injectable ones, may require additional pre-approval before the insurance company will pay for them.

Understanding and working within the guidelines of health insurance is complex. Many companies provide members with access to a vast amount of information on secure websites. This information can help members select a doctor or facility and review the drug formulary. But to understand what a covered benefit is, having a live discussion with an insurance representative is the best course of action. If more and more of the health care costs are being pushed to the member, more and more of the "shopping" decision should also be made by the member.

Our personal experience with insurance was dreadful. I did not realize that radiology services, anesthesia treatments, and blood work were all additional expenses under our healthcare plan. When the surgeon's office quoted his fees, I just assumed it included all the moving parts. It did not! My husband also was operated on in numerous states. State laws need to be followed. Also, doctors can only prescribe pain medications in the state they are licensed in. This became an issue when my husband needed refills. His surgery was performed in North Carolina and he recovered in Georgia. When we went for his follow up appointments, we were able to fill his prescriptions at the hospital pharmacy, but this required traveling to another state and facility. By contacting the financial office in each hospital, I was able to set up appointments to talk about current and past due fees owed and gather information for payment plans. I tried to get a better understanding of how this process worked so our bills would not be sent to a collection's office and if I was able to use my HSA or FSA accounts. I prepared myself the best I could for all the paperwork that is generated. Every year you will need to re-meet your deductibles. It is truly never-ending because scans are required every three to six months along with blood work with your specialist. This is if you are considered in remission. Many more tests and procedures will need to be done if you are still dealing with cancer treatments.

Laurie Johnson Todd is an appendix cancer survivor. She is also called the insurance warrior! She has written two books on the appeals process for a patient who was declined surgery through their insurance. To date, she has won 214 appeals. Fifteen years ago, her own CRS/HIPEC surgeries were declined through her insurance. It was considered experimental surgery. The first case she won was her own. She has helped many caregivers and patients overcome the stresses of insurance appeals. Please reach out to her with any questions at www.theinsurancewarrior.com.

Insurance issues are one of the toughest parts of someone getting sick. There is so much information that you need to know. Remember to write your questions down and never be afraid or embarrassed to ask someone to clarify something you don't understand.

# Chapter 9: Getting a Grip and Gaining Perspective

Throughout our journey, I knew I had many questions, but was unsure what they were and how to ask them. I remember watching a movie called *50/50* with my family. It is about a young, healthy, twenty-something man who gets cancer of the spine. It is a very rare form of cancer. He is an avid runner, but since his back is hurting, he decides to see a doctor. After all the tests are finalized, he sits in a room by himself, waiting for the results. The doctor enters and tells him he has cancer. The patient responds, "A tumor? Me? I mean that does not make sense. I don't smoke, I don't drink...I recycle."

I think no matter what, you will always ask, "Why and how did my spouse get this?" You will also have many discussions with your spouse about the choices he made throughout life and if any of them could have impacted him getting cancer. You research family history and the states you lived in, the weather conditions in those states, and the demographics. You begin to look at the ingredients on the back of food containers and check to see what his hair products are made from. These are moments that the two of you will wrack your brain trying to figure out if there was something you could have done differently.

Another part of the movie I found quite incredible was the dynamics between the main character and the people in his life. He and his mom were close, but he did not want her to know everything and he wanted it to be on his terms. His dad had Alzheimer's, so his mom took care of him. He had a girlfriend at the time who did not treat him very well and a best friend who was goofy but loved him a lot. He started seeing a therapist at the request of his oncologist.

His mother would try calling him every day and he would not pick up his phone…typical for a young adult, right? This is a great opportunity to create boundaries. You should try to figure out where each of you stands on this journey. You can ask questions like:

How does he feel?

Ask him if you are helping him with what he needs?

Ask him if you can do something different?

In the movie, his girlfriend would cancel plans last minute and leave him alone as he tried to prepare dinner for the two of them. He would later find out that she was cheating on him.

You could address relationship issues by asking questions like:

Is this relationship what you both want it to be?

Ask if you trust one another with your life?

Ask if you both meet each other's expectations?

His best friend found out about his girlfriend cheating and talked him into them trying to pick up girls by using his cancer diagnosis. He even helped him shave his head. You can ask questions like:

Is the support system you have enough?

Ask if you need simple tasks done?

When he met with his therapist, she was a pretty woman around twenty-seven years old. They both had different expectations of each other. He thought that she should be this old, bald man wearing a sweater vest. She thought that he would be a middle-aged man with a wife and kids. There was not much trust between the two of them during their first few sessions, but they fall in love with each other at the end of the movie. Another question to ask:

Is this the right time for this new relationship?

One of the poignant moments in the movie is when his mother is trying to make him feel better, so she decides to make him a cup of tea. She says, "I'm going to make you some green tea."

Her son says, "Can't you just come and sit down next to me?"

She says, "I heard on the Today show that green tea reduces your risk of cancer by fifteen percent."

He says, "Well, I've already got cancer... sooooooo...."

I love the humor in it. At some of the most difficult times in your life, you can just laugh. I also love how a mother who is feeling so helpless thinks that a cup of tea will solve it all. I love the naivetés and how she wishes she could go back to a simpler time when her son did not have cancer and a cup of tea was all he needed to make him feel better.

You will try many things to help your spouse. You will remember to buy his favorite wine or cook his favorite meal. You will concede to watching many more football games than you did before. There will also be some negative thoughts in your relationship. You will get a little offended when he does not finish all his food from dinner because this round of chemotherapy was harder for him than he had expected. You will ask, "Why am I eating dinner alone tonight while he is sleeping in a recliner?" You will ask him why he does not want to go for dinner for your daughter's birthday. You will feel hurt, alone, and insulted sometimes. You will feel angry and ask yourself what you did to deserve this. You will wonder why you feel this way. You will think you are selfish for thinking this way of a man with stage IV cancer.

You will approach some of these subjects with him, understanding that he is not doing this intentionally. You will hope he is listening to your concerns and he does not think he is inadequate.

Another line from the film I love is this: "You cannot change your situation; the only thing you can change is how you choose to deal with it." This is so true. It was his therapist telling him how to handle his overbearing mom. She said, "If you are not going to be upfront and honest with her, then expect her to continue to be overbearing." The mom stated in the movie, "I want you to know that I smothered him because I love him." Once her son learned how to be more open with her and allowed her to be a part of his life, she backed off and became much more supportive. She was able to love him for who he was and felt included and special. She already had her husband, who was distant due to his disease and did not want to have that relationship with her son. I tried to make the best out of some sticky situations with my husband. I recall one day he hung up the phone with his "boss" who just told him he did not get a bonus this year because his performance goals were too low. My heart sank as I tried to talk with him about how poorly he was being treated and not focus on the bonus issue. I know he gave his all that year and it was a shame the company did not take him having cancer into consideration. I had many more bad days. Some were just bad despite cancer. But even on a really bad day, I still had to play my role as caregiver.

The main character said something interesting in the movie. "Everyone has been saying you will feel better, and not to worry, and this is all fine, and, like, it's not!"

I do not think it is ever fine again! Some days I realized it was not worth saying anything. Positive or negative. Our drives home from chemo were always quiet. You process where you just were for a few hours, who you saw laying curled up with a blanket and a knit hat on, and how you watched many of the patients sip their ginger ale and eat their animal crackers. I think we overdo the positive remarks because it makes us feel better. If we can wish hard enough, we may be able to make it all better.

My favorite scene was with him and his best friend. They had just had some crazy discussions about how his friend does not understand what it is like to have cancer and that he is only using him to pick up girls. They argued about how the main character felt isolated and alone. His friend was drunk, so the main character decided to drive him home. He put him on the sofa and headed into the bathroom to wash his hands. As he looked for the towel to dry his hands, he saw a book on the floor with many pages folded in titled *Facing Cancer Together!*

It is my favorite scene from any movie! It shows the pain we endure every day. The pain from the patient who is feeling hurt, betrayed, and alone. And the pain from the caregiver who is trying their best to understand how to help the person they love.

It makes you both think, "What are the questions and how do I ask them?"

# Chapter 10: How Important Is It to Have a Support System?

Throughout my entire life, I have made great friends. I come from an Italian family, so we are very social and loud and are there for each other during tough times. I have come across a few people who I have happily moved on from. I used to feel bad if I did not get along with everyone. I felt like I needed to prove myself more for them to truly understand me. Then, my husband got cancer. That changed everything for me! I was slowly evolving over the years before his diagnosis but the words "stage IV cancer" really hit home!

The first person I told was our middle daughter. She was twenty-four-years-old and in school to be a chiropractor. I was confused and did not know how to read the medical terms on the papers the doctor gave me. She is a lot like her dad. She does not lead with emotion. She will analyze a situation first and get to a solution just looking at the facts. She said she would have her professors look at the information and get back to me. She said, "Tell dad the truth about what is going on and then we can talk about the research we have done and fill in the gaps later." She also said, "Mom, do not worry about this. We are going to get through this just fine. You need to think about how you are going to help him." She knows I operate purely on emotion. She knows I overthink everything. I needed to hear her say that, and I am thankful she did.

My husband and I spent the rest of that day in a complete daze. He laid down on the sofa when we got home, and I headed to the office to grab a notebook and pen and start looking for as much information as I could on this specific disease.

My son lived in Florida, so I called him that evening. He has always been our wild-child. He was twenty-six and gave us quite a few scares during his childhood. He did always have the sweetest heart, though. He and his dad never argued but did not have much in common. I could tell when I told him the diagnosis, he was devastated. He is a lot more emotional than his sister, so I knew I had to address it differently. He asked if his dad was going to be okay and choked up a few times. He wanted to know about the dates of surgeries so he could take time off work and be there.

Our youngest daughter, who was eighteen, was visiting her boyfriend in New York when we got the news. I called her to let her know. She is a great combination of her siblings. She can be direct and yet compassionate. We cried together. She is my child who truly gets me. She made me laugh too. She has that effect on me! She felt bad that she was out of town and could not be there for us.

After his colonoscopy, we decided to tell our friends in New York. We called them one evening and explained what we were going through. We heard the sadness and concern in their voices.

Next, we told our families. I had a falling-out with my parents that January so my parents were not the first family members to come to mind when my husband was diagnosed. So, I texted my sister. I know that is not acceptable, but I did not know where to begin! She called me and we spoke, cried, and began to put together a plan to help conquer this disease.

She told our parents. They did text me saying how sorry they were. I had a lot of emotions going through me when I got this text. I knew they loved me. I knew they never wanted my husband to die and I knew they wished that argument never happened. But it did, and now he had stage IV cancer. It did not change the hurtful words said before his diagnosis.

One Saturday afternoon, my husband and I were sitting on the couch. We hadn't showered in a few days and were just depressed. Our children came through the front door, opened the blinds, and shut off the TV. They instructed us to go shower and said we were heading to lunch. They told us to stop wallowing. He was already diagnosed, so quit being so negative and enjoy some fresh air. We had not moved from the house for over a week. We were in a downward spiral. They continued to look after us for a few days to make sure we were making progress and didn't wind up back on the sofa feeling defeated. I am grateful for them for being so observant and acting when they knew we needed it.

I only remember having a relationship with my in-laws when I was younger. They are very distant people and have not liked me for many years. Well, now my husband had to tell them he had cancer! He texted his mother and they talked later that evening. He told her his story and she just sat and listened. She offered to tell his dad and other siblings.

Since both families now knew, I decided to post a lengthy message on Facebook to tell our friends. His sister decided to make a post that created drama within the family. It was not the right time or place. My husband and I discussed the situation and felt that they were concerned but that they acted inappropriately. We understood they retaliated based only on not liking me. I feel this is important because I want to address the negativity from family that can still surround you even when you're dealing with a cancer diagnosis.

My parents showed up after my husband's second surgery and we did not talk about what happened in January. We cheered for my husband's eventful recovery instead. My mom made many meals at my house, as most Italian moms will do, to show that they love you. We never really spoke more about it. I believe actions speak louder than words! I truly wanted to see if they were sorry for what they said and see how our relationship through actions would progress.

I started a group text message with 126 of our closest friends and family. Every week, I would send them an update on him. I also sent them updates every time he had an appointment or procedure done. I bought a picture frame that is linked to an email address so he could receive pictures and inspirational quotes from anyone who wanted to share. It made him happy seeing pictures of when he coached our daughters' softball teams and pictures of our friends and their families.

I also joined two Facebook support groups specific to my husband's appendix cancer. They are very instrumental in helping me navigate this disease. They are called ACPMP Appendix Cancer Support Group, and PMP Pals Network. A nurse navigator can help you find many online support groups or a local support group if that fits your needs.

The surgery date for HIPEC was approaching. We had everything in order. There would be a lot of family and friends attending. I knew it would be a long day. I also knew I would have to make sure to keep the peace between both families. My friends stayed for a few days. My parents stayed the entire time with us and drove us back to Georgia when he was released. My kids, their significant others, sister and brother in law stayed about a week before they had to return to school and work. His mother and two siblings visited him for a few days after surgery when he was still in the hospital.

There was a moment I recall that his mother pulled me on the side and asked if I could help her. It was not something she felt comfortable asking her boys. I thought for a moment how desperate she must have been knowing I was the only person that she could ask for help. I did leave the hospital to get her what she needed and then came back to continue to care for her son. I love how life happens. I did not think after my husband's surgery that I would have much interaction with his family. I know they were there to visit with him. I honestly did not know how I would feel talking to them and prayed many times to not say anything I would later regret. I kept in contact with my sister-in-law through the weekly updates.

When my husband received his first NED after six months, I sent out my message! Everyone was so happy and so thankful and appreciated the great news. His sister did not answer me back. She sent him a message saying congratulations. From that day on, I never heard from her. I had realized the only reason why they communicated with me throughout his surgery and recovery was because he could not message them himself. You think that sickness changes everything. You think it will wash away the past and maybe you can start fresh. If the same people before diagnosis choose to be disrespectful after diagnosis, then nothing will change, not even with cancer!

I spoke with my sister every day and her family housed us many times for appointments and procedures. We would celebrate after appointments by heading to our favorite diner for lunch. Our out-of-state friends sent many messages and cards. It showed how much they cared for us and that they were cheering us on every step of the way. One sent a blanket for him to use at the hospital after his surgery and six lottery tickets to celebrate after his successful chemotherapy treatments. We enjoyed walking in the house after chemo treatments to scratch off a lottery ticket and see if we won anything. My parents spent many weeks at our house making sure our kids were taken care of and that our household was run efficiently. Their actions truly spoke louder than their words. I watched as they were trying to develop a relationship with my husband and rebuild ours. I am not fully healed, but I can no longer sense the black cloud over us anymore. As weird as this may sound, I believe this cancer journey allowed my parents to heal our relationship.

My youngest daughter has a boyfriend who decided to move from New York and attend his senior year of high school in Georgia. He was such a big help during this difficult time. They took over all the household responsibilities and stepped up during the holidays to make sure the house was completely decorated. I believe God places people in your life when you need them. They allowed us to continue with everyday life by helping when or wherever we needed it.

A support group comes in all shapes and sizes. It can be people like family and friends', places like an online support group, or things like fluffy blankets and lottery tickets. Some will truly want to help, and others will just create chaos. Rely on those that are willing to assist you throughout your journey.

Check out some other resources that may help:

- Supporting Spouses of Loved Ones with Cancer on Facebook
- **www.Neverendingcaregiving.com**
- **www.rarediseases.info.nih.gov**
- www.ACPMP.org
- www.Cancer.net
- www.cancer.org
- www.carcinoid.org
- www.hipectreatment.com

# Chapter 11: A New Normal

When your spouse first gets diagnosed, you have a million things running through your mind. You are thinking about how you will get through the next few months, but you never really think about what life will be like if he gets better or if he stays sick or even if he dies. You just trudge through every day because living in the moment is what you need to do to survive.

You have completed all the doctor's visits, all the testing, and all the surgeries. He is now getting scans every six months. He found out he does not need the other six rounds of chemotherapy that he originally thought he would. He is looking to go back to work full-time, something he was not able to do for the last three months. So, now what happens? You just lived the last ten months taking care of your spouse with cancer. He is now able to start back to his normal life. What do *you* do? Everyone said it will be great when he gets cured and you could go back to normal, but no one ever told you about this new normal.

Since my husband has always been so healthy before cancer, I never worried about him being sick. He was the type of guy who had never taken a sick day in thirty-five years. During this cancer journey, I had seen him projectile vomit and assisted him with enemas. If you think childbirth takes away your dignity, say hello to cancer!! Now, I know in my logical brain he is better, but how do I convince my anxiety-ridden-self that he truly is.

I sometimes reminisce about when my husband went away to college. I missed him so much. In the summer months when he was home and before he would leave my house at night, we would talk about how easier our life would be when we did not have to say goodbye every night. We dated for six years before he proposed.

When we got married, we decided to start a family quickly. We did not consider how expensive this might be. Nine months later, we had our son. Life changed for sure...*a new normal* going from a couple to a family of three. Two years later, our daughter was born. Again, *a new normal.*

My husband finished his MBA and was offered a job in New York. His salary doubled and it was a smart career choice, so we packed up and moved our family. We purchased a house on his lunch break because houses were being sold within twenty-four hours after they are listed…*another new normal.*

Now we were parents to two children and owned a home in New York. What just happened? It's all good, right? We were finally doing better financially and were in a brand-new, beautiful town. What else could we ask for?

Well, three months after we settled in, surprise! I was pregnant again. Nine months later, I give birth to this precious baby girl. I was now twenty-nine years old, my husband was thirty-four. Did anyone ever tell you two kids are the right amount because you have enough hands to hold them with? They never quite tell you what to do with the third...oh, well*, a new normal.*

Life was great. Our house was the one on the block that other families visited. We had end-of-year parties where the teachers from their elementary school would come join in the fun. We ran the fall festival at their middle school, and I was PTA president for a few years. We hosted exchange students for two full years and taught all our kids, including the exchange students, how to drive. It seemed like *a new normal* was happening all the time.

You can see that life takes many twists and turns, and yet, we always seem to adjust. But what should I expect from this *new normal* after cancer? Should I expect everything to go back to what it was before? Well, what I learned about life is that you want to evolve. I do not want to be that same twenty-nine-year-old, somewhat-financially-stable girl at forty-seven. I learned so much from *my new normal* along the way that it would be a shame if it stopped now. Sure, I worried about my husband starting back to work full-time. I even took a first-day picture of him and posted on Facebook that it was his first day of preschool. Sure, I ask him more frequently how he is feeling. If he spends longer than normal in the bathroom, I am knocking on the door to make sure everything is alright.

With it now being a year out from surgery, I can say that we make a lot more time for each other. We enjoy the moments we share together, the new memories we build, and forget about the small stuff that just now seems so trivial. The sun shines brighter now! We also appreciate the people who have stood by our side and have reevaluated past relationships that just were too draining.

We grow every time we are put in a different situation. You must try to find a reason to laugh and roll with the punches. This situation will be no different.

Just remember to get lots of rest, though; all these new normals can be exhausting!

# Chapter 12: Where Do I Get the Strength to Take Care of Myself?

After looking at my past, I think I have always been a caregiver. Even when I was young and did not know, I had those tendencies.

When I was in my thirties, my grandmother was diagnosed with pancreatic cancer. We were all devastated. She was already in her eighties but had been perfectly healthy her entire life. Her children and grandchildren all gathered and made a schedule. It included who would be there to feed her, bathe her, and sit with her. She was in her bedroom in the back of the house, withering away. She weighed under eighty pounds. I brought my youngest daughter in from New York with me and stayed at my parents to try to help whenever needed. I stayed for over two weeks until she passed away. I was not as instrumental as my other cousins who lived locally, but I tried to share in the responsibilities.

Then just a few years ago, late one Friday night, we got a phone call from our friend saying his wife was in the ER. She had fallen down their basement steps and broke her leg. Since she was the one who handled all the household responsibilities, I knew she would be worried about how things around her house were going to get done. She had lots of family support but many of them had to juggle full-time jobs and family life of their own. Her husband tried to balance house, family, work, and taking care of her. I visited her in the hospital daily, and when she was transferred to a facility for physical therapy, I made sure she was sticking to her program. I went to their house a few times a week to make meals for her family, clean her house, and do laundry. They had been friends of ours for so many years, but I still knew she would never ask me to help. I knew I had to just show up and look around and begin doing what had to be done. I think I knew what she needed, and I tried to meet those needs. We definitely had many laughs and also cried many tears throughout her journey but our friendship grew stronger.

Years later, my newly met friend who had just gone through a difficult HIPEC procedure was able to move out of the ICU to a room. There were complications and they were able to stop the bleeding! Many surgeons and staff helped her fight for her life. Her family and friends were all praying that she would pull through. My support came in the form of starting a prayer circle on Facebook and continuing to visit her when my husband was recovering.

In these instances, what always kept me going was feeling what it would be like if the tables were turned. Would I be able to ask someone for help? Probably not. And if I did, what would I even ask them to do? My heart always went out to the patient who was feeling vulnerable but knew they could not do it alone.

I also realized how important it was to find my own caregiver! It is nice to schedule a massage, get your nails done, or even get your hair cut. It is better to have someone you can confide in no matter what time of day. *My sister was my caregiver*! I knew early on that she would be my rock. She helped me research, plan, organize, and follow through on everything I said I needed to do. She let me stay accountable for all my actions but also told me when I needed to cut myself some slack because I was being too hard on myself. She checked on me every day by sending me texts or calling me on the phone. She always had the kindest words to say and she listened to me cry, laugh and vent. Most importantly, she was honest with me throughout the whole journey.

I feel my words will resonate with most because when you are feeling overwhelmed, you cannot be specific about your needs. I look at this process as taking a step back and seeing what the patient needs. That is how you can best assist them.

I think you as the caregiver also must step back and allow yourself some space to think more clearly. The more specific you can be, the more help you will receive. The hardest part is trying to figure out what you need. I often asked myself,

Do I need help prepping for meals for the week all day on Sunday?

Would I need a few hours after dinner every night to straighten and clean up the house?

Can I designate Tuesday nights as laundry night and ask for help then?

Can Saturday be the day to mow the lawn and rake leaves?

Can I see who can sit with my spouse while I take our son to baseball practice on Wednesday and Friday nights?

Can I ask friends and family to cook for us two days a week?

Can I ask his friend to sit with him and watch football while I take a hot bath?

The answer to all these questions is YES!

So, you still ask, how do I get the strength to take care of myself?

Well the answer is, you already have the strength within, you just must ask for what you want and when you need it!

# Chapter 13: How Do I Handle the Most Difficult Days?

I have a few words of wisdom that I learned to live by and would love to share what helped me so much throughout my journey.

**\*\* Always leave people better than you found them**

Taking care of a loved one is not for the faint at heart. It is a full-time job. When you are not caring for their needs, other things need to be tended to. Some examples are researching, calling, emailing, documenting, and chauffeuring. Many emotions will surface, and you will need to talk about them with your therapist, your support group, or your caregiver. You will do your best! There will be days where you are still in your pajamas and you did not complete one item on your list. There will be days that you cried and could not get out of bed. There will be days you finished the grocery shopping, laundry, and cleaned your car and it is only 4pm.

So, stay in those pajamas, call your therapist, and cry when you need to!

But remember, just by choosing to help them, *you left them better than you found them.*

**\*\*Someone can love you with their feelings and still not know how to love you with their actions.**

I know I love my husband, but how do I show him I love him? The caregiver role takes on a whole new meaning when you must show your love through actions rather than your feelings. You tell your spouse every night before you go to bed that you love them. I know you mean it, but is it just part of your routine? Did you show them enough times throughout that day so that they felt it? This crazy journey allows you to be open in many ways. You think throughout your marriage you had articulated how much you love him. You think about him every time you purchased a Christmas or birthday present for him. You always asked him how he felt about traveling to Colorado or New York City before you booked the airfare. Isn't that loving him correctly through your actions?

You need to reevaluate what this meant once they get diagnosed. You want desperately to think you had been doing it correctly all these years. You realize there were issues in your life where you had doubted your husband. You took what he said with a grain of salt because sometimes he was not very transparent. You allowed yourself to think this type of behavior was okay because he had let you down before. With a cancer diagnosis now in hand, how do you trust yourself to make the best decisions for his life? You did not trust him fully just a few hours before diagnosis. Am I the right person to make these important calls about *his* life?

You look deep within yourself and pray for many weeks. You try to process how exactly you could help him through this. How could you not create more pain and hurt for him? Is this the time to truly see your differences? Is this when you should be exploring this area of your relationship? You will decide you need to come full circle with all the hurt, pain, and rejection you had felt from him for years. You make a conscious decision that helping to save his life was much more important to you then questioning the times he arrived home late from work. Yes, it is a conscious decision. You sometimes lose your way in a relationship long before they are diagnosed. You've convinced yourself that asking him his opinion on travel plans was an acceptable way to show him you love him. You agree, it is a considerate and helpful way to operate, but is this how you want to take care of him? You feel he deserves better! You feel you can show him you can love him better than that!

It is hard to bury pieces of your past, but you have much more room for new and exciting adventures once you get rid of them. This road is difficult enough not having all your baggage. Take the time to learn about what you feel is important throughout this journey and then begin to focus on *how to love them correctly with your actions.*

\*\*Many patients with appendix cancer do not look sick. They sometimes get overlooked and people make light of a very serious disease. Many caregivers can relate to these points because we are sometimes forgotten for what we go through.

Here's to the people who:

- **Have symptoms you cannot see**. We suffer from the heartache we feel for our loved one. We are anxious wondering if they will be okay, and we struggle with sleep deprivation because we make sure they are comfortable throughout the night. (We still must make sure we get in our well needed rest. Wear headphones to bed or listen to music to fall asleep more comfortably.)
- **Have extreme pain but can function.** Our hearts and minds are pained by knowing every day we must be there to make sure they get everything that they deserve and pray that it will be enough. (We need to nourish our body and mind by eating foods with antioxidants and exercising regularly.)
- **Have many types of illnesses and hide them well**. We hide our sadness, depression, and our anxiety because the focus is on the patient. Our loved

one has enough to deal with. (We need to make sure we are taking our medications and vitamins so we can continue to be healthy for them)

- **Don't look sick from the outside**. We do not look tired or overwhelmed. We are just trying to manage two lives instead of one. (We need to keep our doctors' appointments too.)
- **Have flare-ups.** Our flare-ups happen, but they are not the priority. Our loved one always comes first. (We need to keep a daily journal of how we feel)
- **Fight a daily battle that no one knows**. We fight our daily battles in silence because we are supposed to be the strong ones. (Talk, vent, and curse to our caregiver)

*You got this!*

**\*\*Your current situation is never your final destination.**

In going through this process, you may feel like you are stuck. Time continues to move forward, but here you are in the same spot. Many months go by where you have only gotten bad news. You must stay in your current situation throughout that time. Eventually, one decision will lead to another, and, before you know it, you will be onto the next chapter. Staying in the moment for a while is not always a bad thing. The longer we are at a standstill, the more time we must deal with the issues at hand and make more confident decisions. Remember, you need to allow yourself the time to learn and grow, and then you will appreciate that final destination even more.

**\*\*"It's not my full story, it's just a chapter."** This is what my husband would say throughout this journey. He would say that he had enough great memories and experiences to fill an entire book. He would say cancer will only be a chapter, *the smallest one,* in his book of life!

Remember to find the moments that make that difficult day more enjoyable!

Some extra resources:
- The National Alliance for Caregiving
- Cancer Caregiving

- Cancer Experience Registry/ Caregiver
- Cancer Support Community Helpline 888-793-9355 and **www.cancersupportcommunity.org**
- Cancer Support Community Affiliates and Support Groups for Caregivers
- American Cancer Society- Caregivers Page
- RAISE Family Caregivers Act

# Chapter 14: Your Quality of Life

Did you ever hear anyone say that cancer changed their lives for the good? I have heard many say it made them become a nicer person. They did not sweat the small stuff as much. They appreciated the sunshine more. They spent more time with their family and less time at work.

Stuart Scott, an ESPN anchor, died from appendix cancer in 2015. He said, "Every day, I am reminded that our life's journey is really about the people who touch us." That is profound in so many ways. I have kept so many great relationships throughout my life. I want to be a better person because the people I surround myself with are incredible human beings. They give me the strength and courage to move throughout life. They sympathize with me when I have failed, and they help celebrate me when I succeed! They remind me to take pride in who I am but never be afraid to laugh at myself.

Do not take yourself so seriously. I have been fortunate to have many great role models. I also learned at a young age that you want to be respectful of your relationships. They are never guaranteed. I cannot understand when people say that their marriage, or their relationship with their parents, or kids should be easy. What have we ever done in life that had been easy and yet rewarding at the same time? Your good relationships are that way because you **care**. You put the effort into making them good and that is the reward, you get to experience what it is like to have relationships that touch your life!

I met a woman at an appendix cancer conference who runs one of the support groups I participate in. Her husband is an appendix cancer survivor and she is his primary caregiver for many years. I asked why she has both caregivers and patients on the same site. I am involved with some who are just for spouses and caretakers, not the patients. She said that, in her experience, the caregivers are all about the *care* for their loved one. If they were separated, it would be detrimental to both. The caregiver would not know what could happen from other patients' perspectives and being together meant they could pick up on the warning signs and follow other patients from diagnosis to recovery. I like that answer! I do believe it is all about your spouse's care and what better way to keep on top of it then to hear from other cancer patients!

Stuart Scott's next quote talks about his stage: "I never ask what stage I am in. I have not wanted to know. It will not change anything to me. All I know is that it would cause more worry and a higher degree of freak-out. Stage I, II, or VIII, it does not matter. I am trying to fight it the best I can." It is hard for us to help our loved ones when we do not know all the facts. We still need to consider the patient's rights and not overstep. It is up to us to just find another way to offer our support.

He also said that during a workout, "It feels good to be winded, having trouble breathing, chest hurts…I am alive!" Oh, the simple pleasures! Who knew working out could bring someone so much happiness? Something we typically take for granted breathes new life into him. It must be scary when you think any moment can be your last breath.

Another one of his quotes says, "When you die, it does not mean you lose to cancer. You beat cancer by how you live, why you live, and in the manner in which you live." We chose to not lose to cancer either! Even though my husband did not die and is still NED, it does not mean cancer will not come back. All the tests and procedures he has just means it is not present for now. Some patients go ten years to then head down this road again. Some get cured and new cancer arises. We showed up to beat cancer at every chemotherapy appointment. We started a tradition. On his off weeks of chemo when he was feeling a bit better, we would shop for shirts that we labeled "chemo fun shirts." Even though there is nothing fun about chemo, we wanted to share a laugh or a smile whenever it was possible. They were always a button-down shirt with crazy designs on them. Some were Hawaiian and some were Disney-themed.

We documented a lot with photos, even though we were not in the selfie mood. We made sure we got many pictures together and many of him alone. We made sure to take them with our kids, pets, family, and friends. We celebrated every small event and spent as much time together as we could. It did not matter where we were at; it just mattered that we were together. We talked about his retirement and our future as if nothing changed and continued to share our dreams and goals for the future.

I love my husband very much, but to be honest, I never once said I wished I was the one to have gotten cancer. I often wondered what it would be like if I was the patient. I thought about how my husband would choose to take care of me.

Stuart Scott had lots of family support from his fiancée and children. He spoke highly of how his crew at ESPN had taken great care of him. This last quote sums up how I feel a patient thinks of their caregiver: "So live. *Live!* Fight like hell. And when you get too tired to fight, then lay down and rest and let somebody else fight for you."

# About the Author

Tracy Sparks has dedicated her adult life to helping others. She always puts everyone's interests above her own. This passion started with Tracy's leadership positions on educational and sports league boards while living in Corning, New York. Her approach to writing this book was formulated from a long history of providing unpaid service to the local community, schools, and athletic organizations.

She has helped coordinate benefits for cancer patients in her community and many individuals with rare diseases. She has been a part of fundraising campaigns for start-up organizations. She launched an educational indoor recess program for elementary schools. She has served as a volunteer by being a PTA president, secretary, and treasurer in a local middle school for five years.

She was a food coordinator and staff member in a local youth group retreat for over fifteen years. She was a Girl Scout Troop Leader and a Boy Scout Den Leader for eight years. Tracy and her family have been a part of the Red Cross Kids for over ten years, where they visited nursing homes, cooked meals for the needy, and sang Christmas carols to local veterans during the holidays.

Tracy has been recognized through the American Red Cross Association for her work with military families by receiving The Real Heroes Military Award. She has participated in many appendix cancer symposiums since her husband's diagnosis in 2018. Because of her consistent sacrifices and dedication to providing exceptional service and care, she is now able to apply it in this proven methodology of caregiving to her spouse with stage IV cancer.

# Thank You

If you purchased this book, I am sorry that you are faced with taking care of a loved one who is sick. I am sorry that your life will be turned upside down. I am sorry that you will cry every day and most days feel useless and defeated.

I am sorry we met through these circumstances, but I welcome you with open arms! I hope this book provides you with some knowledge, some laughs, and some peace of mind.

I am offering a free thirty-minute class on the never-ending cycle to caregiving. Please visit my site at [www.neverendingcaregiving.com](www.neverendingcaregiving.com) and enter code FREE to get started.

www.ingramcontent.com/pod-product-compliance
Lightning Source LLC
Chambersburg PA
CBHW070417220526
45466CB00004B/1446